CW01072785

Paleo Diet for Strength

Delicious Paleo Diet Plan, Recipes and Cookbook Designed to Support the Specific Needs of Strength Athletes and Bodybuilders (Food for Fitness Series)

Lars Andersen

Published by Nordic Standard Publishing

Atlanta, Georgia USA

ISBN 978-1-484145-21-0

9 781484 145210 >

All Rights Reserved

No part of this book may be reproduced or transmitted for resale or use by any party other than the individual purchaser who is the sole authorized user of this information. Purchaser is authorized to use any of the information in this publication for his or her own use only. All other reproduction or transmission, or any form or by any means, electronic or mechanical, including photocopying, recording or by any informational storage or retrieval system, is prohibited without express written permission from the author.

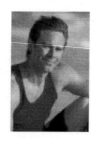

Lars Andersen

Copyright © 2012 Lars Andersen

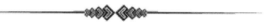

What Our Readers Are Saying

"Finally a way to tailor the Paleo diet to meet my specific training needs - two thumbs up"

★★★★★ **Gordon Haugen (Berkshire, MA)**

"This is exactly the type of book I'd been waiting and it did not disappoint. No more boring cans of tuna for me!"

★★★★★ **Bruce Taylor (Evans, WV)**

"Delicious. Simple. Effective. Deliciously simple and effective in fact!"

★★★★☆ **Brian Irvin (Lockney, TX)**

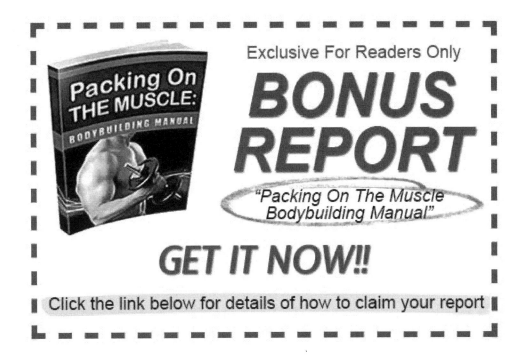

Exclusive Bonus Download: Packing on the Muscle: Bodybuilding Manual

How To Quickly Pack On Swelling Muscles and Explode Your Physique In a Matter of Minutes a Day Without The Use of Drugs or SURGERY! Learn the secrets in using your own body weight and the law of gravity to INCREASE your muscle mass as you strip away the unwanted fat.

Everyone has a routine; whether it's getting up and going to work, or the way you get ready for bed. A body building routine has to be drafted and thoroughly planned out. Everything from eating habits to how many exercises are performed, and even resting time.

Here are some tips:

You have to make sure you adjust your protein-rich diet as well as your eating habit. Small light meals instead of 3 full-course meals a day would be a normal approach to building your body.

Not only is meal a factor in a body building routine, but the exercise is also a factor. You need strength training excercises that involve both compound and isolated movements.

Nutrition provides a great role in your routine because of the calorie intake. You require more calories than an average person with the same weight due to the protein and energy it takes to excercise.

Your muscle growth occurs only after the exercise, during rest. Without proper rest, your muscles cannot have the opporitunity to heal or increase in size

This is your quick guide to that summer beach body you've always wanted. This manual will cover:

- Body Building Diet Tips
- Body Building Routines
- Body Building Supplements
- Body Building Workouts
- Building Muscle the Natural Way
- Healthy Body Building Nutrition Tips
- How to Build Strength
- Losing Body Fat the Natural Way
- Weight Training Routines
- Weight Training Tips
- And Much Much MORE!!!

<u>Go to the end of this book for the download link for this Bonus!</u>

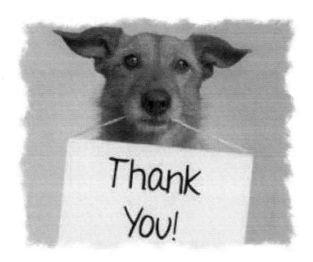

Thank you for downloading my book. Please REVIEW this book on Amazon. I need your feedback to make the next version better. Thank you so much!

Books by Lars Andersen

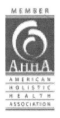

Table of Contents

Disclaimer

While all attempts have been made to provide effective, verifiable information in this Book, neither the Author nor Publisher assumes any responsibility for errors, inaccuracies, or omissions. Any slights of people or organizations are unintentional.

This Book is not a source of medical information, and it should not be regarded as such. This publication is designed to provide accurate and authoritative information in regard to the subject matter covered. It is sold with the understanding that the publisher is not engaged in rendering a medical service. As with any medical advice, the reader is strongly encouraged to seek professional medical advice before taking action.

Paleo and High Protein Diet for Strength Training and Muscle Building

"One should eat to live, not live to eat" – Benjamin Franklin

The current US Department of Agriculture (USDA) healthy eating guidelines promote a balanced daily diet consisting of 60 percent carbohydrates, 30 percent fats, and 10 percent protein. Switching from USDA recommendations to a Paleo diet will generally lead to an increase in your overall protein and fat intake and a drop in your overall carbohydrate intake. However, your main sources of carbohydrates will be fruits and vegetables, meaning that you will gain a plentiful supply of healthful micro-nutrients, and your main sources of protein and fats will be lean meats with low levels of saturated fat, and fish with high levels of omega-3 essential fatty acids.

The recommended amount of protein in a healthy diet is calculated on the basis of an average of 0.9 grams of protein per 2 pounds of body weight per day. If you are in regular training with the goal of building muscle, you may need to increase your daily intake slightly, but this would be to no more than an average of 1.2 to 1.7 grams per 2 pounds of body weight per day. This means that a pound of extra protein in your daily diet will *not* equate to a pound of extra muscle on your biceps, but it could equate to an extra pound of unwanted weight around your waistline!

Steak has long been heralded as the food of choice for bodybuilders, and with good reason. Meat is a good source of protein, and protein plays an important role in tissue growth and repair. However, steak is not necessarily the best source of protein available and excessive amounts of protein from any source do not need to be consumed in order to build muscle.

Protein is present in your muscles and also in your bones, skin, nails, hair, tendons and arteries. All body proteins are continually being broken down and replaced, and it's through your diet that the protein needed to replenish stores is found. However, not all dietary sources of protein are equal and no natural food is pure protein, unlike the many dietary sources of pure carbohydrate or fat. The quality of the protein you consume is of far greater importance in terms of body building than the quantity, and a mix of different sources is the best way to ensure you gain the optimal quantities of essential amino acids. All proteins are made up of amino acids, some of which can be produced naturally by your body, but others can only be sourced through your diet.

All of the essential amino acids are present to some degree in most protein foods but to be fully utilized by your body, they must be present in optimal proportions. For example, if you eat a protein food that contains half of the ideal proportions of one of the essential amino acids, your body can only use half of the other essential amino acids present. The other half would be wasted or used by your body as an energy source in the absence of carbohydrates for fuel.

Paleo Protein

The Paleo diet can be summed up in one simple rule of thumb proposed by Paleo advocates; "If it's in a box, you shouldn't be eating it." Paleo is the common name given to the Paleolithic diet, so named because of its similarities to the diet of our hunter-gatherer ancestors some 2.5 million years ago in the Paleolithic Era. In essence, it's a diet that revolves around eating foods which occur naturally and avoiding foods which would be unrecognizable to a Paleolithic caveman! Meat *would* have been a staple in Paleolithic times but grain-fed meat *would not.* Paleo sources of meat protein are quality sources, including the following:

Beef – with the exception of fiber, beef contains most of the nutrients your body needs:

- Calcium- essential for strong bones and teeth, and plays an important role in nerve transmission and muscle functions.
- Vitamin C – needed to make collagen, a protein essential for healthy gums, teeth, bones, cartilage and skin. Also aids the absorption of iron from plant food and is an important antioxidant. Antioxidants protect against free radicals, potentially harmful chemicals which are formed by your body as a by-product of its metabolic processes.
- Folate – needed for the formation of proteins in the body.
- Iron – an essential component of hemoglobin, the oxygen carrying pigment in red blood cells, and also important in energy metabolism.
- Iodine – vital for the production of thyroid hormones which govern the efficiency of converting food into energy.
- Manganese – a vital component of many enzymes involved in energy production.
- Zinc – vital for normal growth and development, and plays an important role in the functioning of the immune system.
- Selenium – an antioxidant which protects against free radical damage.
- Chromium – monitors blood sugar levels and stimulates glucose uptake in cells. Also helps to control fat and cholesterol levels in the blood.
- Fluoride – plays a role in protecting tooth enamel against the acids which may cause decay.
- Silicon – required for strong, flexible joints and connective tissues.

Organic, grass-fed beef provides far greater health benefits than grain-fed beef but the overall vitamin and mineral content depends on the quality of the soil grazed. Lean beef contains less than five percent fat, half of which is saturated fat.

Lamb – provides a rich source of protein, B vitamins, zinc and iron.

Pork – one of the leanest meat sources of protein; lower in fat than beef and lamb. A useful source of zinc and iron and an excellent source of B vitamins:

- B vitamins – play an important role in releasing energy from food.
- Vitamin B12 – essential for all growth and division of cells, and for red cell formation.

Offal – ox liver and calves' liver are rich sources of easily absorbed iron. Also:

- Vitamin A – needed for normal cell division and growth, and plays an important role in maintaining the mucous membranes of the respiratory, digestive and urinary tracts.
- Vitamin B12

Kidneys also provide a rich source of B12 and both liver and kidney are low in fat.

Game and Game Birds – provide excellent sources of protein, with a much lower fat content than domesticated animals such as chicken. This category includes sources such as venison, rabbit, wild boar and pheasant. They offer a rich source of B vitamins and iron, also:

- Potassium – essential for the transmission of all nerve impulses, and works in conjunction with sodium to maintain a healthy fluid and electrolyte balance within the cells. Electrolytes are charged particles that circulate in the blood, helping to regulate the body's fluid balance.
- Phosphorus – essential for the absorption of many nutrients, and plays a vital role in the release of energy in cells.

Wild game, when available, represents a chemical free source of protein compared to farmed game, but sources must always be sustainable.

Fish – all forms of fish provide excellent sources of protein, however, wild varieties offer healthier options than farmed versions. This also applies to **seafood**, with organic sources of crab, oysters, shrimp, scallops, lobster mussels and clams representing healthier choices.

- **Oysters** – excellent source of zinc and copper, needed for healthy bone and connective tissue growth. Copper also helps the body to absorb iron from food and is present in many enzymes which protect against free radical damage.
- **Mussels** – rich source of iron and iodine.
- **Scallops** – rich source of selenium.
- **Crab** – good source of potassium and zinc; also contains magnesium, which assists in nerve impulses and is important for muscle contraction.
- **Shrimps** – rich source of iodine; also useful source of selenium and calcium.
- **Clams** – excellent source of iron and useful source of zinc.

Eggs – omega-3 enriched eggs offer an excellent source of protein and healthy fat; a large egg contains around 6-8 grams of protein and 5-7 grams of fat, around 2 grams of which is saturated fat.

However, it's recommended that no more than six eggs should be consumed per week due to the high cholesterol content. A rich source of:

- Vitamin B12
- Choline (in yolks) – aids the transport of cholesterol in the blood and plays an important role in fat metabolism.

Hemp – provides a good source of protein, a healthy balance of omega-3 and omega-6 essential fatty acids, and contains many B vitamins, vitamin A, calcium and iron. Also:

- Vitamin D – needed to absorb calcium and phosphorus.
- Vitamin E – an important antioxidant.
- Sodium – essential for nerve and muscle function, and works in conjunction with potassium to regulate the body's fluid balance.
- And dietary fiber.

Green leafy vegetables – greens provide a good source of plant protein along with many other health benefits:

- **Beet greens** – the leafy tops of beets contain calcium, iron and beta-carotene, a powerful antioxidant. Research has also found that consuming beets on a regular basis can enhance an athlete's tolerance to high-intensity exercise.
- **Collard greens** – a good source of omega-3 essential fatty acids which have anti-inflammatory properties.
- **Lettuce** – a good source of vitamin C, beta-carotene, folate, calcium and iron.
- **Mustard greens** – an excellent source of antioxidant vitamins A, C, E, and vitamin K which plays an essential role in the formation of certain proteins. Also contains carotenes and flavonoids which are powerful antioxidants, and calcium, iron, magnesium, potassium, zinc, selenium and manganese.
- **Swiss chard** – a rich source of vitamin A, C and K, B vitamins, omega-3 fatty acids, and a number of antioxidants and flavonoids. Also contains copper, calcium, sodium, potassium, iron, manganese and phosphorus.
- **Turnip greens** – a rich source of beta-carotene, vitamin C, and a useful source of folate.
- **Spinach** – a rich source of carotenoids, including antioxidants beta-carotene and lutein. Also contains vitamin C and potassium.

Cruciferous vegetables

- **Cabbage** - rich source of vitamin C, vitamin K, and a good source of vitamin E, potassium and beta-carotene. Vitamin K is essential in the formation of many proteins - the body's building blocks - and vitamin E has an important role to play in preventing free radical damage.
- **Broccoli** - another rich source of vitamin C. Broccoli also contains beta-carotene, iron and potassium, and is high in bioflavonoids and other antioxidants. Iron is essential for the production of hemoglobin, the oxygen carrying pigment in red blood cells, and myoglobin, a similar pigment which stores oxygen in your muscles.
- **Kale** - a good source of iron, calcium, vitamin C and beta-carotene.
- **Cauliflower** – a rich source of vitamin C.
- **Rutabaga** – a good source of vitamin A and iron.

- **Kohlrabi** – a good source of vitamin C, calcium, phosphorus and iron.
- **Watercress** – rich source of vitamin C, beta-carotene and iron.

Protein is essentially the body's muscle-builder but adding protein to your diet does not in itself build muscle in body building terms. It is resistance training and progressive overload that builds muscle, however consuming moderate amounts of quality protein can help to promote tissue growth and repair, thereby aiding your recovery after each training session. To train effectively you need to fuel your body with carbohydrates.

Paleo Carbohydrates

Paleo carbohydrate sources are mainly fruits and vegetables. Carbohydrates can be split into two main categories: simple carbohydrates or **sugars**, and complex carbohydrates or **starches**. Starches provide a much slower release of energy compared to sugars, making them the preferred source of fuel for athletes in training. The natural sugar content of most fruits means they must be consumed in moderation to avoid sugar "spikes" and "crashes" whereas the majority of vegetables can be consumed on an "all you can eat" basis.

Good sources include:

- **Cassava** – a good source of naturally "starchy" carbohydrate. Also provides calcium, iron, manganese, phosphorus, potassium, B vitamins, vitamin C and dietary fiber. Cassava flour is gluten-free.
- **Taro root** – a starchy vegetable offering a rich source of potassium, and a useful source of calcium, vitamins C and E, B vitamins, manganese, magnesium and copper. Taro leaves are also relatively high in protein.
- **Plantains** – a good low sugar source of starchy carbohydrate, also an excellent source of potassium and dietary fiber, and a useful source of vitamins A and C.
- **Yam** – a good source of vitamin B6, vitamin C, potassium and manganese.
- **White potatoes** – a good source of starchy carbohydrate, protein and fiber. They also provide vitamin C and potassium.
- **Sweet potatoes** – a good source of vitamin B6, vitamin C, vitamin D, iron, magnesium, potassium and beta-carotene.
- **Squash** – a good source of vitamins C and A, and also a useful source of calcium and iron.

In moderation, the following fruits also provide a good source of carbohydrate:

- **Strawberries** - a rich source of vitamin C and also an aid to the absorption of iron from vegetables.
- **Pears** - a good source of vitamin C, potassium, pectin and bioflavonoids. Pectin provides fiber, and bioflavonoids are powerful antioxidants.
- **Mangoes** - a good source of vitamin C and beta-carotene.
- **Bananas** - a rich source of potassium.
- **Apple** – offers a small amount of vitamin C.
- **Peach** – a good source of vitamins A and C.
- **Blueberries** - often described as "the ultimate brain food," blueberries have an antioxidant content of around five times higher than other fruits and vegetables.

Both fruits and vegetables provide a healthful source of carbohydrates for energy but the added fiber content of vegetables helps to slow the absorption of sugar and thereby a slower and steadier release of energy is provided. Dark green leafy vegetables are nutritionally dense, making them an ideal source of energy to fuel strength and muscle building training sessions. All carbohydrates are converted into glucose and glycogen before they can be used to fuel everyday activities and exercise. While training, the working muscles are fuelled by glucose in the blood, and by glycogen from stores in the liver and in the muscles. Glucose and glycogen are inter-convertible. When the body has a sufficient supply of glucose, carbohydrates are converted to glycogen and stored, but if glucose is in short supply, glycogen is converted to glucose ready for use. Your body can only store a limited amount of glycogen, with the muscles able to store enough for up to around two hours of intense exercise. After exercising, your body's ability to store glycogen is elevated. This period of around 30 minutes is known as the "glycogen window" and consuming appropriate foods in this window helps replenish glycogen stores, promote muscle repair and restoration, and thereby aid recovery after a long or intense training session.

Paleo Fats

Not all fats are equal. Like carbohydrates, fats also provide energy. In fact, fats yield nine calories per gram compared to only four calories per gram for carbohydrates. However, fat is a much slower source of energy so when you are training hard, your body relies on your glycogen stores to fuel your performance by providing a faster release of energy. All carbohydrates are converted to glycogen and stored in your body. During sub-maximal training sessions, your body aims to conserve as much of its glycogen reserves as possible by using some of its fat stores for energy instead.

Good quality fat sources in a Paleo diet are the saturated fats provided by grass-fed meat and the fat provided by organic eggs. The preferred cooking fats are tallow, lard, grass-fed butter, ghee, coconut oil, palm oil and occasionally olive oil, although processed oils should be avoided whenever possible and used for dressing foods rather than cooking foods. Some oils contain high levels of omega-6 fatty acids which can cause an inflammatory response in your body. For this reason, most nut and seed oils should be used sparingly. Macadamia nuts offer the lowest levels of omega-6 but alternatives include flax seed oil (linseed oil), walnut oil, canola and avocado oil. Avocados themselves are a rich source of healthy fat, with one fruit containing as many as 400 healthful calories.

Your body can make its own fat from excess carbohydrates and protein in your diet but it cannot manufacture certain essential unsaturated fats, meaning that the foods you eat are your body's only supply. The essential fatty acids are omega-3, found in green leafy vegetables and some vegetable oils, and omega-6, found in vegetable oils such as olive oil and sunflower oil. Creating a healthy omega-6 and omega-3 balance with a ratio of 2:1 or 1:1 brings optimum benefits in terms of overall health and wellbeing. Fats act as a carrier for fat-soluble vitamins, including vitamins A, D, K, and E, and they provide insulation and protection for your body.

Many nuts and seeds provide excellent sources of fat and also protein. Good choices include:

- **Flax seeds** - also known as linseeds, provide a good source of protein and are high in omega-3 essential fatty acids. They also contain B vitamins which are involved in the release of energy from food.
- **Pumpkin seeds** – a rich source of protein and fat along with numerous vitamins and minerals including B vitamins, vitamin E, copper, manganese, potassium, calcium, magnesium, iron, zinc and selenium. Copper is present in many enzymes which protect against free radicals and helps the body to absorb iron from food.
- **Sunflower seeds** – provide protein along with vitamin E, selenium, magnesium and copper.

- **Almonds** – provide protein along with calcium, magnesium, potassium, vitamin E and other antioxidants.
- **Cashews** – a good source of protein and rich in iron, phosphorus, selenium, zinc and magnesium.
- **Walnuts** – provide protein and also a rich source of omega-3 fatty acids.

Adding oils to raw foods such as salad leaves, or to foods after cooking as a dressing, is a practical way to boost your healthy fat intake. Popular choices include olive oil and coconut oil. The "healthy" saturated fat content of coconut oil provides energy-giving calories and many other health benefits including anti-inflammatory properties.

Paleo Power

The quality foods you eat provide quality fuel for your body, allowing you to put in a quality effort in every training session. Paleo "purists" eat only foods which can be hunted, fished or gathered. Foods include meat, offal, seafood, eggs, insects, fruits, nuts, seeds, vegetables, mushrooms, herbs and spices. Excluded foods include grains, legumes – beans and peanuts – dairy products, refined sugar, salt and processed oils. However, other Paleo-based diets include "modern" foods which were not available to our cavemen ancestors but support the macronutrient composition of a Paleolithic diet none-the-less. These foods include milk and dairy products, rice, potatoes and some processed oils such as olive oil or canola oil.

If you choose to include some dairy products in your Paleo diet, a green smoothie made with green leafy vegetables, fruit, and milk or yogurt can provide a convenient and nutritionally dense post-training recovery booster. Milk contains whey protein which is fast-acting and helps to reduce the effects of muscle damage immediately after an intense training session, and casein protein which is slow-acting and helps to continue the repair process long afterwards.

Cutting all "modern" foodstuffs from your diet, including all forms of grain as well as highly processed convenience foods, leaves a diet of all natural foodstuffs which can be summarized as follows:

- **Meat** – grass-fed rather than grain-fed animal sources.
- **Fowl** – chicken, turkey, duck, and game birds.
- **Fish** – wild fish rather than farmed fish as the latter can contain unhealthy levels of mercury and other toxins.
- **Eggs** – organic, free range and ideally omega-3 enriched.
- **Vegetables** – excluding modern farmed varieties.
- **Oils** – any natural source such as coconut oil, walnut oil, or avocado oil.
- **Fruits** – berries in particular and other fruits in moderation.
- **Nuts** – excluding peanuts.
- **Tubers** – sweet potatoes and yams in particular.

There is no *one* Paleo diet, and it's important to note that a Paleo-based diet is not necessarily a "low-carb diet" as such. Some hunter-gatherer populations would have survived and thrived on a low-carb diet; others would have lived equally well on a high-carb diet of fish, tubers, and coconut. An important element of all Paleo-based diets is that locally sourced organic produce should make up the bulk of your daily food intake whenever possible. However, this can prove expensive in some areas of today's world, so aiming to eat the best quality produce you can afford is an important step in terms of getting the most from a Paleo diet. The key to maximizing your "Paleo power" is eat a diet of *real* foods; quality protein and fat in moderation, unlimited vegetables, limited fruits, and the avoidance of all refined carbohydrates and grains containing gluten.

There's a lot of truth in the old adage, "You are what you eat," and while eating lean meat will not instantly add lean mass to your body, a diet of healthy, organic and natural foods will give you the quality fuel you need to reap quality rewards from your training efforts.

Paleo Recipes - Strength Training

Breakfasts

Orange cake

Preparation time	15 minutes
Ready time	1 hour
Serves	8
Serving quantity/unit	364 G / 13 ounces
Calories	107 Cal
Total Fat	29g
Cholesterol	103mg
Sodium	358mg
Total Carbohydrates	20g
Dietary fibers	5g
Sugars	12g
Protein	12g
Vitamin C	0.13
Vitamin A	0.04
Iron	0.11
Calcium	0.13

Ingredients

- 3 ¼ cups of almond meal
- 1 tsp. of baking powder
- 2 tsps. of cinnamon
- 1 tbsp. of orange grind
- 5 organic eggs, yolks and whites separated
- 4 tbsps. of raw honey
- 3 + 1 tbsps. of coconut oil, melted
- 4 tbsps. of grass-fed milk or almond milk
- ½ cup of orange juice

Method

- Preheat the oven to 350°F.
- Combine the yolks, 3 tablespoons of oil and honey in a large bowl and add the milk.
- Mix flour with baking soda, orange grind and cinnamon and add to the egg mixture.
- Beat the egg whites until stiff and carefully fold them in the cake batter.
- Grease a cake pan with the remaining coconut oil and line it with non-stick baking paper. Pour in the batter and bake for 45 minutes or until a toothpick comes out clean.
- Set aside to cool but turn into a serving plate while still warm. Prick the top of the cake gently with a fork and spoon over the orange juice.

Scrambled eggs with mushrooms and parsley

Preparation time	10 minutes
Ready time	20 minutes
Serves	1
Serving quantity/unit	100 G / 4 ounces
Calories	122 Cal
Total Fat	8.6 g
Cholesterol	247mg
Sodium	391mg
Total Carbohydrates	2g
Dietary fibers	0g
Sugars	2g
Protein	10g
Vitamin C	0.03
Vitamin A	0.09
Iron	0.08
Calcium	0.06

Ingredients

- 6 organic eggs, beaten
- 4 tbsps. of grass-fed milk or almond milk
- 1 cup of mushrooms, chopped
- 1 garlic clove, finely sliced
- 1 tbsp. of parsley, finely sliced
- ½ tbsp. of coconut oil, melted
- ½ tsp. of pepper
- ½ tsp. of salt

Method

- Preheat a non-stick pan.
- Combine the organic eggs, milk and parsley, salt and pepper and mix.
- Pour the oil into the pan, add the mushrooms and cook for 4-5 minutes or until tender.
- Add the egg mixture, cook for half a minute and gently stir with a wooden spoon, folding it over from the pan's edges to center until the organic eggs form creamy curds. Remove from heat and serve.

Coconut mango muffins

Preparation time	15 minutes
Ready time	1 hour
Serves	7
Serving quantity/unit	94 G /3 ounces/2 small muffins
Calories	371 Cal
Total Fat	31 g
Cholesterol	117 mg
Sodium	363 mg
Total Carbohydrates	15 g
Dietary fibers	5g
Sugars	8g
Protein	13g
Vitamin C	0.04
Vitamin A	0.04
Iron	0.12
Calcium	0.12

Ingredients

- 2 ¾ cups of almond meal
- ½ cup of organic coconut flakes
- 2 tbsps. of raw honey
- 3 tbsps. of coconut oil, melted
- 1/3 cup of dried mango
- 5 organic eggs
- 1 tsp. of baking soda

Method

- Preheat the oven to 350°F.
- Combine the yolks, oil and honey in a large bowl.
- Pulse the almond meal and the coconut flakes in a food processor until a fine flour forms.
- Transfer to a bowl, add the baking soda, mix, and combine with the organic egg mixture.
- Slice the dried mango and add to the batter
- Beat the egg whites until stiff and carefully fold them in the cake batter.
- Pour the batter into 14 paper muffin liners and bake for 45 minutes or until a toothpick comes out clean.

Banana smoothie

Preparation time	5 minutes
Ready time	5 minutes
Serves	4
Serving quantity/unit	300 G / 11 ounces
Calories	277 Cal
Total Fat	12 g
Cholesterol	0mg
Sodium	107mg
Total Carbohydrates	42g
Dietary fibers	5g
Sugars	28g
Protein	5g
Vitamin C	0.14
Vitamin A	0.09
Iron	0.06
Calcium	0.04

Ingredients

- 2½ cups of almond milk
- 2 ½ cups of banana
- 6 tbsps. of sunflower seed
- ¼ cup of pecan nuts
- ¼ cup of almonds
- 2 tbsps. of raw honey
- 2 tsps. of cinnamon

Method

- Combine all the ingredients in a food processor and pulse until smooth.

Coconut crepes with fresh fruit and nuts

Preparation time	15 minutes
Ready time	45 minutes
Serves	4
Serving quantity/unit	205 G/7 ounces/2 crepes
Calories	374 Cal
Total Fat	32 g
Cholesterol	205 mg
Sodium	92mg
Total Carbohydrates	16g
Dietary fibers	4g
Sugars	12g
Protein	11g
Vitamin C	0.62
Vitamin A	0.32
Iron	0.14
Calcium	0.07

Ingredients

Crepes:

- 5 organic eggs
- ¾ cup of coconut grass-fed milk or almond milk
- 1/3 cup of almond meal
- 1/3 cup of coconut flakes
- 2 tbsps. of coconut oil
- Serve with:
- 1 cup of strawberries, chopped
- 1 cup of melon, chopped
- 2 tbsps. of pecan nuts, chopped
- 1 tbsp. of raw honey

Method

Crepes:

- Pre-heat a non-stick pan.
- Pulse the coconut flakes and the almond meal in a food processor until very fine flour is formed.
- Combine the eggs, milk, and one tablespoon of oil in a large bowl and mix until the batter is homogenous.
- Add the almond and coconut flour and whisk until the batter is smooth.
- Brush the pan with the remaining coconut oil and pour in ¼ of batter.
- Gently tilt the pan until the surface is evenly covered with batter and cook for 1 or 2 minutes, until golden.
- Turn and cook the other side.
- Serve with the fresh fruit, pecans and honey.

Apple and lemon pancake

Preparation time	10 minutes
Ready time	30 minutes
Serves	4
Serving quantity/unit	116 G / 4 ounces
Calories	323 Cal
Total Fat	25 g
Cholesterol	124mg
Sodium	53mg
Total Carbohydrates	17g
Dietary fibers	5g
Sugars	11g
Protein	12g
Vitamin C	0.06
Vitamin A	0.04
Iron	0.11
Calcium	0.13

Ingredients

- 3 organic eggs
- ¼ cup of whole grass-fed milk or almond milk
- 1 ½ cups of almond meal
- ½ cup of unsweetened apple sauce
- 2 tbsps. of lemon
- 1 ½ tbsps. of raw honey
- 1 tbsp. of coconut oil, melted

Method

- Pre-heat a non-stick pan.
- Combine the eggs, milk, almond flour, applesauce, lemon and honey in a large bowl mixing until the batter is smooth.
- Brush the pan with the coconut oil and pour in ¼ to 1/3 batter, cook for 2 or 3minutes, until bubbles burst on the surface, turn and cook the other side for 1 minute or until golden.
- Serve immediately.

Banana coconut bread

Preparation time	15 minutes
Ready time	55 minutes
Serves	6
Serving quantity/unit	114 G / 4 ounces
Calories	336 Cal
Total Fat	22 g
Cholesterol	82 mg
Sodium	357 mg
Total Carbohydrates	32 g
Dietary fibers	5g
Sugars	22 g
Protein	8g
Vitamin C	0.06
Vitamin A	0.03
Iron	0.07
Calcium	0.07

Ingredients

- 1 ¼ cups of almond flour
- ¼ cup of coconut flour
- 1 tsp. of baking soda
- 2 bananas
- 1/3 cup of raw honey
- ¼ cup of coconut oil, melted
- 3 organic eggs

Method

- Preheat oven to 350F.
- Mash the bananas.
- Combine the almond meal, coconut flour and baking soda in a food processor.
- Add the mashed banana, raw honey, oil and eggs to the flour mixture and pulse until the batter is homogenous.
- Scoop batter into a small loaf pan and bake for 35-40 minutes or until a toothpick comes out clean.

Snacks

Mexican tomato salsa

Preparation time	15 minutes
Ready time	40 minutes
Serves	4
Serving quantity/unit	250 G / 9 ounces
Calories	99 Cal
Total Fat	4 g
Cholesterol	0 mg
Sodium	325 mg
Total Carbohydrates	15 g
Dietary fibers	4 g
Sugars	8 g
Protein	2g
Vitamin C	1.06
Vitamin A	1.43
Iron	0.04
Calcium	0.04

Ingredients

Tomato salsa:

- 4 tomatoes, halved
- 1 ½ onions, quartered
- 2 fresh jalapeno peppers
- 4 garlic cloves, unpeeled
- 1 tbsp. of olive oil
- 1 tbsp. of lime juice

- ½ tsp. of salt
- ½ tsp. of pepper
- 1 ½ tbsps. of fresh cilantro, finely chopped
- Serve with:
- 2 carrots, cut into strips
- 1 celery stalk, cut into strips
- 1 red bell pepper, cut into strips

Method

- Preheat the oven to 350F.
- Place the tomatoes, onion, jalapeno peppers and garlic cloves in an oven safe dish and roast the vegetables for 15-20 minutes or until tender.
- Remove from oven and let cool.
- Peel the garlic and remove the stem of the jalapeno peppers.
- Combine the roasted vegetables in a food processor and pulse until they are coarsely chopped.
- Transfer to a bowl and add the salt, pepper and lime juice and cilantro. Stir until well blended
- Serve the with the carrot, bell pepper and celery strips.

Melon, banana and strawberry smoothie with kale

Preparation time	5 minutes
Ready time	5 minutes
Serves	4
Serving quantity/unit	260 G / 9 ounces
Calories	113 Cal
Total Fat	1 g
Cholesterol	0 mg
Sodium	34 mg
Total Carbohydrates	27 g
Dietary fibers	4g
Sugars	17 g
Protein	3g
Vitamin C	2.15
Vitamin A	1.83
Iron	0.07
Calcium	0.07

Ingredients

- 2 cups of strawberries
- 3 cups of melon
- 1 cup of banana
- 2 cups of kale

Method

- Combine all the ingredients in a food processor and pulse until smooth.

Grilled pineapple with cinnamon and cashews

Preparation time	5 minutes
Ready time	20 minutes
Serves	4
Serving quantity/unit	132 G/5 ounces/2 pineapple slices
Calories	140 Cal
Total Fat	4 g
Cholesterol	0 mg
Sodium	3 mg
Total Carbohydrates	27 g
Dietary fibers	3g
Sugars	20g
Protein	2g
Vitamin C	0.89
Vitamin A	0.01
Iron	0.05
Calcium	0.03

Ingredients

- 8 fresh raw pineapple slices, peeled
- 2 tsp. of cinnamon
- 2 tbsp. of raw honey
- 2 tbsp. of water
- 4 tbsp. of cashews

Method

- Preheat an electric griller or a non-stick pan.
- Stir the honey, water and cinnamon in a small bowl until well blended. You can microwave this mixture for 15-20 seconds before serving.
- Grill the pineapple for two or three minutes on each side.
- Serve two pineapple slices topped with raw honey mixture and one tablespoon of cashews per person.

Apple cinnamon squares

Preparation time	20 minutes
Ready time	40 minutes
Serves	8
Serving quantity/unit	55 G / 2 ounces/1 square
Calories	168 Cal
Total Fat	13 g
Cholesterol	21 mg
Sodium	12 mg
Total Carbohydrates	12 g
Dietary fibers	2g
Sugars	7g
Protein	4g
Vitamin C	0.01
Vitamin A	0.01
Iron	0.06
Calcium	0.05

Ingredients

- ¾ cup of almonds
- ¾ cup of dried coconut chips
- 1 tbsp. of flax seed
- 3 tbsps. of water
- 2 tbsps. of raw honey
- 3 tbsps. of almond butter
- 1 tbsp. of grass-fed milk or almond milk
- 1 organic egg
- 1 cup of apple
- 1 tsp. of cinnamon

Method

- Preheat oven to 350F.
- Pulse the flax seeds in a food processor until grind, transfer into a small bowl and add two tablespoons of water. Set aside.
- Pulse the almonds and coconut chips in a food processor until a fine flour forms.
- Combine the honey, almond butter, egg, flax seed mixture, milk and cinnamon in a large bowl and mix until well blended.
- Add the almond mixture and mix. Finally, fold in the apple.
- Press the batter into a small square/rectangular baking pan previously lined with non-stick baking paper. Bake for 15-20 minutes. Let cool and cut into squares.

Sweet potato chips

Preparation time	15 minutes
Ready time	1 hour
Serves	4
Serving quantity/unit	120 G / 4 ounces
Calories	133 Cal
Total Fat	4 g
Cholesterol	0 mg
Sodium	332 mg
Total Carbohydrates	24 g
Dietary fibers	4g
Sugars	7g
Protein	2g
Vitamin C	0.37
Vitamin A	4.38
Iron	0.04
Calcium	0.04

Ingredients

- 4 sweet potatoes, thinly sliced
- 1 tbsp. of olive oil
- ½ tsp. of salt

Method

- Preheat oven to 250F and line baking sheets with non-stick baking paper.
- Put the sweet potato slices, olive oil, and salt in a large bowl and toss to combine.
- Lay the sweet potato pieces in the baking sheets and bake for 45 minutes or until crisp.

Cucumber sandwiches

Preparation time	15 minutes
Ready time	1 hour
Serves	4
Serving quantity/unit	120 G / 4 ounces
Calories	133 Cal
Total Fat	4 g
Cholesterol	0 mg
Sodium	332 mg
Total Carbohydrates	24 g
Dietary fibers	4g
Sugars	7g
Protein	2g
Vitamin C	0.37
Vitamin A	4.38
Iron	0.04
Calcium	0.04

Ingredients

- 2 large cucumbers
- 8 ham slices
- 2 tbsps. of mayonnaise

Method

- Slice the cucumbers.
- Cut the ham slices into squares proportional to the cucumber slices. Set aside.
- Spread a bit of mayonnaise into half of the cucumber slices and top each of them with a ham square. Use the other half of the cucumber slices to close the sandwiches.

Apricot cookies

Preparation time	15 minutes
Ready time	30 minutes
Serves	5
Serving quantity/unit	40 G / 1 ounce
Calories	143 Cal
Total Fat	10 g
Cholesterol	0 mg
Sodium	22 mg
Total Carbohydrates	10 g
Dietary fibers	2g
Sugars	8 g
Protein	5g
Vitamin C	0
Vitamin A	0.01
Iron	0.03
Calcium	0.03

Ingredients

- 2/3 cup of almond meal flour
- 2 organic egg whites
- 1 tbsp. of coconut oil, melted
- 1 tbsp. of raw honey
- 3 tbsps. of dried apricots, cut into small pieces

Method

- Preheat the oven to 350F.
- Line a baking sheet with non-stick baking paper.
- In a food processor combine the flour, egg whites, coconut oil and honey until smooth.
- Transfer to a mixing bowl and fold in the apricot pieces.
- Scoop tablespoons of dough onto the prepared baking sheets and flatten each dough portion a little with your hands.
- Cook for 8-10 minutes or until golden.
- Remove from heat and let cool.

Bell pepper and carrot omelet muffin

Preparation time	15 minutes
Ready time	40 minutes
Serves	4
Serving quantity/unit	100 G / 4 ounces
Calories	95 Cal
Total Fat	6g
Cholesterol	206 mg
Sodium	379 mg
Total Carbohydrates	3 g
Dietary fibers	1g
Sugars	2g
Protein	8g
Vitamin C	0.42
Vitamin A	0.41
Iron	0.06
Calcium	0.05

Ingredients

- 5 organic eggs, beaten
- 3 tbsps. of grass-fed milk or almond milk
- 4 tbsps. of green bell pepper, chopped
- 4 tbsps. of red bell pepper, chopped
- 4 tbsps. of grated carrot, chopped
- 2 tbsps. of onion, chopped
- 2 tsps. of parsley
- ½ tsp. of salt
- ½ tsp. of pepper
- ¼ tsp. of chili powder

Method

- Preheat the oven to 350F.
- Stir the organic eggs, milk, salt, pepper and parsley in a large bowl until well blended.
- Prepare the filling combining the bell peppers, carrot and onion in a bowl.
- Place a small amount of filling into the bottom of muffin paper liners, pour organic egg mixture into each cup of and bake for 20-25 minutes or until muffins are light golden brown.

Lunches

Guacamole and shrimp rolls

Preparation time	30 minutes
Ready time	50 minutes
Serves	4
Serving quantity/unit	425 G / 15 ounces
Calories	267 Cal
Total Fat	16 g
Cholesterol	124 mg
Sodium	155 mg
Total Carbohydrates	20 g
Dietary fibers	7 g
Sugars	6 g
Protein	17g
Vitamin C	0.42
Vitamin A	0.13
Iron	0.18
Calcium	0.08

Ingredients

- 3 cucumbers
- 9 ounces of wild shrimp, peeled
- 1 ½ avocados
- 3 garlic clove, finely chopped
- 1 tbsp. of olive oil
- 1 onion, finely chopped
- 3 tbsps. of lemon juice

- 1 tbsp. of fresh coriander
- 1 tomato
- ½ tsp. of salt
- ½ tsp. of pepper

Method

- To prepare the guacamole, halve and pit the whole avocado and scoop out the flesh from the peal of both avocados.
- Reserve the peel and transfer the flesh to a bowl and mash with a fork.
- Add the garlic, onion, cilantro, lemon, a little salt, and the coriander and mash some more. Cover and refrigerate until serve.
- Heat the oil in a non-stick skillet and cook the shrimp with a pinch of salt and pepper until fully cooked. Let cool and chop.
- Thinly slice the cucumbers lengthwise with a vegetable peeler or mandolin.
- Spread a small amount of the guacamole on one side of each cucumber slice and top with the shrimp
- Roll up the cucumber slices and serve.

Roast beef cuts with sweet potato chips

Preparation time	45 minutes
Ready time	6 hours
Serves	4
Serving quantity/unit	300 G / 11 ounces
Calories	446 Cal
Total Fat	24 g
Cholesterol	70 mg
Sodium	1018 mg
Total Carbohydrates	31 g
Dietary fibers	6g
Sugars	9 g
Protein	25g
Vitamin C	0.5
Vitamin A	4.43
Iron	0.19
Calcium	0.09

Ingredients

Roast beef:

- 1 pound of grass fed boneless rump roast
- 1 tsp. of salt
- 3 garlic cloves, halved
- ¼ cup of wine of your choice
- 1 tbsp. of classic Dijon mustard (unsweetened)
- 1 ½ onions, sliced
- 2 tbsps. of rosemary
- 1 tbsp. of crumbled bay leaves
- 2 tbsps. of parsley, finely chopped
- 1 ½ + ½ tbsps. of olive oil

Sweet potato chips:

- 4 sweet potatoes, thinly sliced
- ½ tsp. of salt
- ½ tsp. of pepper

Method

Roast beef:

- Place the meat in a large bowl and make small incisions around the roast with a sharp kitchen knife, insert a garlic piece into each incision. Set aside.
- In a small bowl, combine the wine, mustard, rosemary, parsley.
- Marinate the meat on the wine mixture for at least 3 hours in the refrigerator.
- Remove the meat from the refrigerator around 30 minutes before cooking.
- Preheat oven to 375F.
- Brush an oven-safe dish with half a tablespoon of olive oil and arrange the onion slices evenly on the bottom of the dish.
- Spread the remaining olive oil around the meat.
- Transfer the meat and juices to the prepared oven-safe dish, fatty side up, and sprinkle with salt.
- Cover with aluminum foil and roast for 25-30 minutes.
- Remove the foil, lower the heat to 250F and cook for further one hour or until meat is cooked to desired doneness, basting occasionally with the juices.
- Let cool and slice with a sharp knife.

Sweet potato chips:

- Preheat oven to 250F and line baking sheets with non-stick baking paper.
- Put the sweet potato slices, olive oil, and salt in a large bowl and toss to combine.
- Lay the sweet potato pieces in the baking sheets and bake for 45 minutes or until crisp.

Cauliflower rice and egg salad

Preparation time	5 minutes
Ready time	5 minutes
Serves	1
Serving quantity/unit	370 G / 13 ounces
Calories	222 Cal
Total Fat	11 g
Cholesterol	143 mg
Sodium	866 mg
Total Carbohydrates	20 g
Dietary fibers	8 g
Sugars	10 g
Protein	15 g
Vitamin C	2.34
Vitamin A	1.15
Iron	0.12
Calcium	0.1

Ingredients

- 1 large cauliflower head
- 1 cup of grass-fed ham, cubed
- 3 organic eggs, beaten
- 3 tbsps. of grass-fed milk or almond milk
- 1 cup of carrot
- 1 red bell pepper
- 1 onion, finely chopped
- 1 tablespoon of olive oil
- ½ tsp. of salt
- ½ tsp. of pepper
- ½ tsp. of cumin
- 1 tbsp. of parsley

Method

- Place the cauliflower in a food processor and pulse until it is the size of rice.
- Transfer to a microwave-safe dish, season with salt and cumin, cover and microwave on high in periods of 5 minutes, stirring and verifying the cauliflower consistency between each period, until tender.
- Transfer to a large mixing bowl and set aside.
- Combine the eggs, milk and pepper in a mixing bowl.
- Heat the oil in a non-stick skillet, add the egg mixture, cook for half a minute and stir with a wooden spoon, folding it over from the pan's edges to the middle until the egg is dryer and fully cooked. Remove from heat and cut into smaller pieces if necessary.
- Add the onion, carrot, ham and egg to the cauliflower and toss to combine.

Halibut patties

Preparation time	25 minutes
Ready time	45 minutes
Serves	4
Serving quantity/unit	260 G / 9 ounces
Calories	388 Cal
Total Fat	17 g
Cholesterol	61 mg
Sodium	417 mg
Total Carbohydrates	38 g
Dietary fibers	8 g
Sugars	11 g
Protein	24g
Vitamin C	0.59
Vitamin A	4.9
Iron	0.21
Calcium	0.17

Ingredients

- 2 ½ cups of sweet potato, cubed
- 7 ounces of wild halibut
- 2 garlic cloves
- 1 onion
- 3 tbsps. of Parsley
- 1 tbsp. of oregano

- 2 tbsps. of capers
- ½ tsp. of salt
- ½ tsp. of black pepper
- 1 organic egg
- ¾ cup of almond flour
- ¼ cup of cashews
- 2 tbsps. of lemon juice

Method

- In a large pan, bring to a boil enough water to cook the halibut.
- Add the fish and cook for 15-20 minutes or until the fish is fully cooked.
- Remove from heat, let cool and drain the water. Shred the fish and set aside.
- Preheat oven to 350F.
- Microwave sweet potatoes on High for 5 minutes or until just tender. Transfer to a mixing bowl and mash with a fork. Add the fish and remaining ingredients, except for the flour, and stir to combine.
- Divide into 12 portions and shape each one into a patty with your hands.
- Coat the patties with the almond flour, remove the excess and lay them on baking sheets lines with non-stick baking paper.
- Bake for 10-15 minutes, flip and cook for further 10-15 minutes or until fully cooked.

Chicken and mango salad

Preparation time	20 minutes
Ready time	20 minutes
Serves	4
Serving quantity/unit	420 G / 15 ounces
Calories	394 Cal
Total Fat	23 g
Cholesterol	49 mg
Sodium	380 mg
Total Carbohydrates	29 g
Dietary fibers	6g
Sugars	20 g
Protein	23 g
Vitamin C	0.84
Vitamin A	1.12
Iron	0.17
Calcium	0.11

Ingredients

- 9 ounces of grass-fed chicken breasts
- 1 ½ tsps. of curry powder
- ½ tsp. of salt
- 2 mangoes
- ½ onion, finely chopped
- 1 cucumber, cubed
- 3 tbsps. of fresh cilantro
- 6 cups of lettuce, shredded
- 6 cups of spinach
- ½ cup of pecan nuts
- 3 tbsps. of lime juice
- 2 tbsps. of sunflower oil
- 1 tbsp. of olive oil
- ½ tsp. of pepper

Method

- Season the chicken breasts with salt and curry, and cook them on a non-stick skillet with olive oil. Let cool and cut into small pieces.
- Stir the sunflower oil, lime juice, pepper, and cilantro in a small bowl until well blended. Set aside
- Place the greens in a large bowl, add the onion, nuts, cucumber, mango and chicken. Toss to combine.
- Add the lime dressing immediately before serving.

Stuffed red cabbage cups

Preparation time	25 minutes
Ready time	40 minutes
Serves	4
Serving quantity/unit	400 G / 14 ounces /2 cups
Calories	317 Cal
Total Fat	12 g
Cholesterol	42 mg
Sodium	292 mg
Total Carbohydrates	28 g
Dietary fibers	8 g
Sugars	11 g
Protein	26g
Vitamin C	2.63
Vitamin A	2.51
Iron	0.21
Calcium	0.16

Ingredients

- 2 cans of tuna in water
- 1 onion, finely chopped
- 4 tbsps. of dill, finely chopped
- 2 yellow bell peppers, chopped
- 2 cups of broccoli, finely chopped
- 2 cups of carrot, cubed
- 2 tbsps. of sunflower seed
- 2 tbsps. of olive oil
- 6 tbsps. of mayonnaise
- 8 large red cabbage leaves

Method

- Drain the water from the tuna cans.
- Heat the olive oil in a skillet, add the onion and cook until translucent.
- Add the carrot, broccoli and bell pepper and cook for 7-10 minutes stirring. Let cool and transfer to a mixing bowl.
- Add the dill, sunflower oil, mayonnaise and stir to combine.
- Scoop a portion of this mixture into each cabbage leaf and serve.

Honey lemon chicken skewers with grilled vegetables

Preparation time	30 minutes
Ready time	10h
Serves	1
Serving quantity/unit	396 G / 14 ounces
Calories	331 Cal
Total Fat	14 g
Cholesterol	54 mg
Sodium	649 mg
Total Carbohydrates	32 g
Dietary fibers	5 g
Sugars	25 g
Protein	23 g
Vitamin C	1.95
Vitamin A	0.64
Iron	0.13
Calcium	0.07

Ingredients

Chicken skewers:

- 9 ounces of grass-fed chicken breast, cubed
- 3 tbsps. of sunflower oil
- ¼ cup of lemon juice
- ¼ cup of raw honey
- 4 garlic cloves, finely chopped
- ½ tsp. of salt
- ½ tsp. of pepper
- 1 tbsp. of oregano

Grilled vegetables:

- 4 tomatoes, halved
- 2 zucchinis, cut into thick slices
- 2 green bell peppers, cut for skewering
- ½ tsp. of salt
- 1 tbsp. of oregano

Method

Chicken skewers:

- In a large bowl, combine the oil, lemon juice, honey, garlic, salt, pepper and oregano, whisk. Add the chicken and marinate overnight in the refrigerator.
- Preheat the grill.
- Remove the chicken from the refrigerator.
- Thread meat pieces onto metal skewers and grill for 5 minutes on each side, or until the meat is fully cooked.

Grilled vegetables:

- Preheat grill.
- Sprinkle oregano and a little bit of salt on the cut side of tomatoes.
- Alternate the zucchini and bell pepper on a metal skewer and season with the remaining salt, grill for 2-3 minutes on each side.
- Place the tomatoes with the cut side up on the grill and cook for 7-9 minutes. Turn and cook the other side for further 7-9 minutes.

Dinner recipes

Shrimp and squid skewers with tomato and cucumber salad

Preparation time	30 minutes
Ready time	50 minutes
Serves	4
Serving quantity/unit	590 G / 21 ounces
Calories	303 Cal
Total Fat	13 g
Cholesterol	266 mg
Sodium	764 mg
Total Carbohydrates	25 g
Dietary fibers	6 g
Sugars	11 g
Protein	25g
Vitamin C	2.05
Vitamin A	0.71
Iron	0.24
Calcium	0.13

Ingredients

Shrimp and squid skewers:

- ½ pound of wild shrimp
- ½ pound of wild squid, cut for skewering
- 2 green bell peppers, cut for skewering
- 2 onions, cut for skewering
- 2 zucchinis, cut into thick slices
- 4 garlic cloves, finely chopped

- ½ tsp. of chili powder
- 3 tbsps. of parsley, finely chopped
- 3 tbsps. of lemon juice
- 2 tbsps. of clarified butter, melted
- ¼ tsp. of salt
- ½ tsp. of white pepper

Salad:

- 4 tomatoes, cubed
- 2 cucumbers, cubed
- ½ cup of black olives, sliced
- 1 tbsp. of olive oil
- ½ tsp. of salt
- ½ tsp. of pepper

Method

Shrimp and squid skewers:

- Preheat grill.
- In a small bowl combine the butter, lemon juice, garlic, parsley, chili, salt and pepper.
- Alternate shrimp, squid pieces and vegetables on metal skewers and grill for 5 minutes on each side, or until the shrimp is fully cooked, brushing each side with the butter mixture.

Salad:

- Prepare the salad combining all the salad ingredients in a large mixing bowl.

Fish balls with tomato salsa and roasted eggplant

Preparation time	30 minutes
Ready time	5 hours
Serves	1
Serving quantity/unit	600 G / 21 ounces
Calories	509 Cal
Total Fat	27 g
Cholesterol	144 mg
Sodium	729 mg
Total Carbohydrates	37 g
Dietary fibers	15g
Sugars	15 g
Protein	38g
Vitamin C	1.06
Vitamin A	0.33
Iron	0.18
Calcium	0.14

Ingredients

Fish balls:

- 1 pound of wild cod
- 1 cup of cauliflower, chopped
- 1 onion, chopped
- 3 garlic cloves, chopped
- 1 ½ tbsps. of olive oil
- 3 tbsps. of parsley, chopped
- ½ tsp. of salt
- ½ tsp. of chili Powder
- 3 tbsps. of lemon juice
- 2 organic eggs
- ½ cup of almond flour
- 4 lemon wedges

Tomato salsa:

- 4 tomatoes, halved
- 1 ½ onions, quartered
- 2 Fresh Jalapeno peppers, whole
- 4 garlic cloves, whole
- 1 tbsp. of olive oil
- 1 tbsp. of lime juice
- ¼ tsp. of salt
- 1 tbsp. of fresh cilantro

Roasted eggplant:

- 2 organic eggplants, sliced lengthwise
- 2 tbsps. of olive oil
- 3 tbsps. of lemon juice
- ¼ tsp. of salt
- ½ tsp. of pepper

Method

Fish balls:

- Preheat oven to 350F.
- In a large pan, bring to a boil enough water to cook the cod and cauliflower.
- Add the fish and cook for 15-20 minutes or until it is fully cooked.
- Remove from heat, and carefully remove the fish from the water with a metal spatula and set aside.
- Add the cauliflower to the fish cooking liquid. Return to heat, bring to a boil and cook the cauliflower for 10 minutes or until tender.
- Shred the fish and transfer to a food processor.
- Add the cauliflower and the remaining ingredients (except for the lemon wedges and almond flour) and pulse until they are finely chopped and with a moldable consistency.
- Divide into small portions and shape each one into a ball with your hands.
- Coat the balls with the almond flour, remove the excess and lay them on baking sheets lined with non-stick baking paper.
- Cook in the oven for 35-45 minutes, or until they turn light golden brown.

Tomato salsa:

- Preheat the oven to 350F.
- Place the tomatoes, onion, jalapeno peppers and garlic cloves in an oven safe dish and roast the vegetables for 15-20 minutes or until tender.
- Remove from oven and let cool.
- Peel the garlic and remove the stem of the jalapeno peppers.
- Combine the roasted vegetables in a food processor and pulse until they are coarsely chopped.
- Transfer to a bowl and add the salt, pepper, lime juice and cilantro. Stir until well blended.

Roasted eggplant:

- Preheat oven to 375F.
- Place the eggplant slices on the oven rack and bake them with an oven baking sheet below, for 20-30 minutes or until tender.
- Transfer into a heat-proof bowl, cover and let cool.
- In a mixing bowl combine the olive oil, lemon juice, salt and pepper.
- Marinate the organic eggplants in this mixture for at least 3 hours.

Crustless Italian sausage quiche

Preparation time	15 minutes
Ready time	50 minutes
Serves	4
Serving quantity/unit	240 G / 8 ounces
Calories	297 Cal
Total Fat	20 g
Cholesterol	286 mg
Sodium	510 mg
Total Carbohydrates	9 g
Dietary fibers	1g
Sugars	7 g
Protein	20g
Vitamin C	0.08
Vitamin A	0.1
Iron	0.14
Calcium	0.13

Ingredients

- 1 onion, chopped
- 2 cups of mushrooms, chopped
- 6 oz./170g of organic Italian sausage, sliced
- ¼ cup of sun dried tomato, chopped
- 6 organic eggs
- 1 cup of grass-fed milk or almond milk
- ½ tsp. of oregano
- ½ tsp. of basil

Method

- Preheat oven to 350F.
- Heat a non-stick skillet, add the sausage and onion and cook for five minutes.
- Add the mushrooms and cook for 10 minutes, add one or two tablespoons of water if necessary.
- Remove from heat, add the tomatoes and stir to combine.
- Combine the organic eggs and milk in a mixing bowl.
- Line an oven-safe dish with non-stick baking paper, distribute the ham mixture evenly in the bottom of the dish and sprinkle with the herbs.
- Pour organic egg mixture on top.
- Bake for 30-35 minutes or until light golden brown.

Zucchini and tuna bake

Preparation time	45 minutes
Ready time	1h30m
Serves	4
Serving quantity/unit	440 G / 15 ounces
Calories	468 Cal
Total Fat	10 g
Cholesterol	36 mg
Sodium	400 mg
Total Carbohydrates	18 g
Dietary fibers	6g
Sugars	7 g
Protein	24 g
Vitamin C	1.39
Vitamin A	1.38
Iron	0.16
Calcium	0.13

Ingredients

- 2 tbsps. of olive oil
- 1 ½ onions, finely chopped
- 2 garlic cloves, finely chopped
- 1 ½ cups of peeled tomatoes, chopped
- 1 cup of carrot, sliced
- 1 celery stalk, sliced
- 1 red bell pepper, chopped
- 2 cans of tuna in water
- 5 cups of zucchini, thinly sliced
- ½ tsp. of salt
- ½ tsp. of pepper
- 1 tbsp. of oregano
- 1 tbsp. of basil
- ½ tbsp. of rosemary

Method

- Preheat oven to 350F.
- Drain the liquid from the tuna cans.
- Heat the oil in a large skillet and cook the onion and garlic until translucent.
- Add the tomatoes, carrot, celery and bell pepper; season with salt, oregano, basil and rosemary. Cook for 10 minutes.
- Add the tuna, stir and cook for 5 minutes, or until the vegetables are tender.
- Arrange two layers of zucchini slices on the bottom of an oven safe dish and top it with half of the tuna mixture.
- Assemble another layer of zucchini slices and spread the other half of the tuna mixture evenly on top.
- Finish with one layer of zucchini slices and sprinkle them with a pinch of salt.
- Bake for 30 to 45 minutes (until the zucchini is cooked and the top layer is golden brown).

Orange and raw honey glazed ham with cauliflower rice

Preparation time	30 minutes
Ready time	2 hours
Serves	4
Serving quantity/unit	428 G / 15 ounces
Calories	347 Cal
Total Fat	11 g
Cholesterol	65 mg
Sodium	1094 mg
Total Carbohydrates	43 g
Dietary fibers	9g
Sugars	29 g
Protein	24g
Vitamin C	2.39
Vitamin A	0.05
Iron	0.16
Calcium	0.12

Ingredients

Ham:

- 1 pound of grass-fed ham, reduced sodium
- ½ cup of fresh orange juice
- 1 sliced orange
- ¼ cup of raw honey
- 1 tbsp. of classic Dijon mustard, unsweetened
- 2 tbsps. of rosemary
- ½ tsp. of cloves
- Cauliflower rice:
- 1 large cauliflower head
- ¼ tsp. of salt
- ½ tsp. of pepper

Method

Ham:

- Preheat oven to 370F.
- Combine the orange juice, honey, mustard and rosemary in a mixing bowl.
- Make small incisions in the ham with a sharp knife and insert the cloves.
- Arrange the orange slices around the ham fixing them with toothpicks.
- Pour over 1/3 of the orange juice mixture and bake for 45-60 minutes, basting frequently with the remaining glaze.
- Cauliflower rice:
- Place the cauliflower in a food processor and pulse until it is the size of rice.
- Transfer to a microwave-safe dish, season with salt and pepper, cover and microwave on high in periods of 5 minutes, stirring and verifying the cauliflower consistency between each period, until tender.

Beef on a bed of onion with roasted sweet potatoes and beets

Preparation time	30 minutes
Ready time	2 hours
Serves	4
Serving quantity/unit	515 G / 18 ounces
Calories	503 Cal
Total Fat	17 g
Cholesterol	57 mg
Sodium	767 mg
Total Carbohydrates	64 g
Dietary fibers	11g
Sugars	27 g
Protein	27g
Vitamin C	0.89
Vitamin A	7.72
Iron	0.26
Calcium	0.13

Ingredients

Grass-fed beef:

- 9 ounces of grass-fed top sirloin steaks
- 4 large onions, sliced
- 2 ½ tbsps. of olive oil
- ½ tsp. of salt
- ½ tsp. of pepper
- ½ tsp. of paprika

Roasted sweet potatoes and beets:

- 4 cups of sweet potatoes, cubed
- 2 cups of beets, cubed
- 1 tbsp. of olive oil
- ½ tsp. of salt
- ½ tsp. of pepper

Method

Grass-fed beef:

- Season the meat with pepper and paprika and set aside.
- Pour the olive oil into a large pot.
- Set the heat to low, add a couple tablespoons of water, and then spread the onion slices evenly on the bottom of the pot.
- Place each steak on top of the onions so that they are not on top of each other.
- Cover the pot and cook for 15 minutes. Turn the steaks and cook the other side for further 15 minutes or until the meat is cooked to desired doneness.
- Roasted sweet potatoes and beets:
- Preheat oven to 300F and line baking sheets with non-stick baking paper.
- Put the sweet potato, beet olive oil, salt and pepper in a large bowl and toss to combine.
- Lay the sweet potato and beet pieces in the baking sheet and bake for 1 hour or until crisp.

Herbed grilled salmon with roasted bell pepper

Preparation time	30 minutes
Ready time	4 hours
Serves	4
Serving quantity/unit	306 G / 11 ounces
Calories	409 Cal
Total Fat	29 g
Cholesterol	71 mg
Sodium	515 mg
Total Carbohydrates	10 g
Dietary fibers	4 g
Sugars	7 g
Protein	27 g
Vitamin C	3.58
Vitamin A	1.06
Iron	0.08
Calcium	0.04

Ingredients

Salmon:

- 1 pound wild salmon
- ½ tsp. of salt
- ½ tbsp. of parsley
- ½ tbsp. of fresh oregano
- ½ tbsp. of fresh basil

Roasted bell pepper:

- 4 large red bell peppers, whole
- 4 tbsps. of olive oil
- 3 tbsps. of apple cider vinegar
- ½ tsp. of black pepper
- ¼ tsp. of salt

Method

Salmon:

- Preheat a non-stick skillet.
- Season the salmon with the salt and herbs and cook it over low heat for 5-7 minutes on each side until it's fully cooked.

Roasted bell pepper:

- Preheat oven to 375F.
- Place the peppers on the oven rack and cook them in the oven, with an oven baking sheet below, for 30-45 minutes or until most of the skin has darkened.
- Transfer into a heat-proof bowl, cover and let cool.
- Peel the peppers removing all the darkened skin. Cut them into strips
- In a mixing bowl combine the olive oil, vinegar, salt and pepper. Marinate the peppers in this mixture for at least 3 hours.

Dessert recipes

Crustless pumpkin pie

Preparation time	10 minutes
Ready time	1 hour
Serves	4
Serving quantity/unit	150 G / 11 ounces
Calories	153 Cal
Total Fat	5 g
Cholesterol	82 mg
Sodium	82 mg
Total Carbohydrates	22 g
Dietary fibers	3 g
Sugars	17 g
Protein	7g
Vitamin C	0.05
Vitamin A	1.94
Iron	0.09
Calcium	0.04

Ingredients

- 1 cup of pumpkin
- 3 tbsps. of blanched almond flour
- 2 organic eggs
- 2 organic egg whites
- 3 tbsps. of raw honey
- 1 tbsp. of pumpkin spice
- ½ cup of almond milk

Method

- Preheat oven to 375F.
- Transfer all the ingredients into a food processor and pulse until it is smooth.
- Pour the mixture onto a pie plate.
- Place the pie plate in a baking pan and fill ¼ of the baking pan with hot water.
- Bake for 45-50 minutes or until a knife inserted in the center comes out clean.

Mango and lemon sorbet

Preparation time	5 minutes
Ready time	3 hours
Serves	4
Serving quantity/unit	170 G / 6 ounces
Calories	89 Cal
Total Fat	0 g
Cholesterol	0 mg
Sodium	4 mg
Total Carbohydrates	24 g
Dietary fibers	2 g
Sugars	21 g
Protein	1 g
Vitamin C	0.5
Vitamin A	0.13
Iron	0.01
Calcium	0.01

Ingredients

- 2 cups of mango, cubed
- 2 tbsps. of raw honey
- 1 cup of ice
- ¼ cup of lemon juice

Method

- Combine all the ingredients in a food processor.
- Transfer to a metal container, cover and freeze for 3-4 hours or until it is hard on the edges and slushy in the middle.

Strawberry lemon cake

Preparation time	20 minutes
Ready time	1h20m
Serves	1
Serving quantity/unit	100 G / 4 ounces
Calories	207 Cal
Total Fat	15 g
Cholesterol	65 mg
Sodium	190 mg
Total Carbohydrates	14 g
Dietary fibers	3g
Sugars	10 g
Protein	7g
Vitamin C	0.33
Vitamin A	0.02
Iron	0.06
Calcium	0.05

Ingredients

- 1 ½ cups of almond flour
- 4 organic eggs
- 2 organic egg whites
- 4 tbsps. of raw honey
- ¼ cup of olive oil
- ½ cup of almond milk
- 3 tbsps. of lemon juice
- 1 tbsp. of lemon rind
- 1 tsp. of baking soda
- 2 cup of strawberries chopped

Method

- Preheat the oven to 350°F.
- Combine the strawberries and three tablespoons of water in a medium saucepan and bring to a simmer.
- Simmer for 10-15 minutes or until the strawberries are soft and the syrup thickens, add the honey, stir and remove from heat. Set aside.
- Combine the yolks, 3 tablespoons of oil, lemon juice and remaining raw honey in a large bowl and add the milk.
- Mix flour with baking soda and lemon grind and add to the egg mixture.
- Beat the egg whites until stiff and carefully fold them in the cake batter.
- Grease a cake pan with the remaining oil and line it with non-stick baking paper.
- Pour in half of the batter and carefully spread the strawberry syrup on top of it.
- Spread the remaining batter evenly on top and bake for 45 minutes or until a toothpick comes out clean.

Coconut and chocolate cupcakes

Preparation time	20 minutes
Ready time	1 hour
Serves	4
Serving quantity/unit	105 G / 4 ounces
Calories	282 Cal
Total Fat	13 g
Cholesterol	205 mg
Sodium	430 mg
Total Carbohydrates	30 g
Dietary fibers	12g
Sugars	11 g
Protein	12g
Vitamin C	0
Vitamin A	0.05
Iron	0.13
Calcium	0.04

Ingredients

- 5 organic eggs, yolks and whites separated
- 6 tbsps. of raw cocoa
- 1 cup of coconut flakes

62

- 2 tbsps. of raw honey
- 1 tbsp. of coconut oil, melted
- 1 tsp. of baking soda

Method

- Preheat the oven to 350°F.
- Combine the yolks, oil and honey in a large bowl.
- Pulse the coconut flakes, cocoa and baking soda in a food processor until a fine flour forms. Add to the organic egg mixture.
- Beat the egg whites until stiff and carefully fold them in the cake batter.
- Pour the batter into paper cupcake liners and bake for 25-30 minutes or until a toothpick comes out clean.

Banana and cherry ice cream

Preparation time	10 minutes
Ready time	8 hours
Serves	4
Serving quantity/unit	180 G / 6 ounces
Calories	227 Cal
Total Fat	11 g
Cholesterol	0 mg
Sodium	2 mg
Total Carbohydrates	35 g
Dietary fibers	5g
Sugars	19 g
Protein	3g
Vitamin C	0.22
Vitamin A	0.02
Iron	0.06
Calcium	0.01

Ingredients

- 4 frozen bananas
- 1 cup of cherries, pitted
- ½ cup of coconut cream

Method

- Place the cherries in a food processor and pulse until coarsely chopped. Transfer to a bowl and set aside.
- Process the bananas and coconut cream in the food processor until the mixture becomes firm and smooth.
- Combine the banana mixture and cherries in a mixing bowl.
- Cover and freeze overnight.

Passion fruit pudding

Preparation time	10 minutes
Ready time	8 hours
Serves	4
Serving quantity/unit	180 G / 6 ounces
Calories	227 Cal
Total Fat	11 g
Cholesterol	0 mg
Sodium	2 mg
Total Carbohydrates	35 g
Dietary fibers	5g
Sugars	19 g
Protein	3g
Vitamin C	0.22
Vitamin A	0.02
Iron	0.06
Calcium	0.01

Ingredients

- 3 organic eggs, beaten
- 1 cup of passion fruit
- 1 cup of coconut cream
- 1 tbsp. of raw honey
- ½ cup of almond milk
- 1 oz./28g of unflavored gelatin

Method

- Place all the ingredients in a food processor and pulse until it is smooth.
- Transfer into pudding dish and refrigerate overnight.

Chocolate mousse

Preparation time	30 minutes
Ready time	5 hours
Serves	6
Serving quantity/unit	70 G / 3 ounces
Calories	242 Cal
Total Fat	14 g
Cholesterol	144 mg
Sodium	78 mg
Total Carbohydrates	23 g
Dietary fibers	1g
Sugars	20 g
Protein	7g
Vitamin C	0
Vitamin A	0.06
Iron	0.09
Calcium	0.09

Ingredients

- 6 oz./200g of organic dark chocolate
- 5 organic eggs, yolks and whites separated
- 1 ½ tbsp. of fresh mint, finely chopped

Method

- Melt the chocolate in a double boiler stirring frequently, until smooth.
- Let cool a little and combine with the yolks in a mixing bowl, stirring vigorously. Add the mint.
- Beat the organic egg whites until stiff and carefully fold them in the chocolate mixture.
- Refrigerate for at least 5 hours before serving.

Exclusive Bonus Download: Packing on the Muscle: Bodybuilding Manual

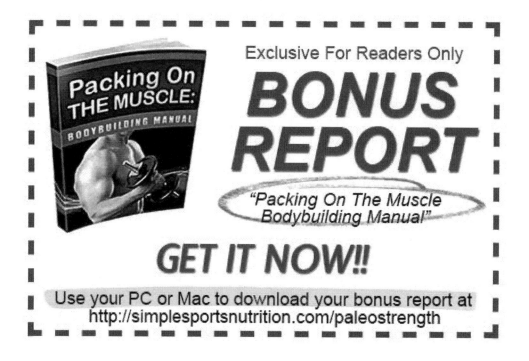

Download your bonus, please visit the download link above from your PC or MAC. To open PDF files, visit http://get.adobe.com/reader/ to download the reader if it's not already installed on your PC or Mac. To open ZIP files, you may need to download WinZip from http://www.winzip.com. This download is for PC or Mac ONLY and might not be downloadable to kindle.

How To Quickly Pack On Swelling Muscles and Explode Your Physique In a Matter of Minutes a Day Without The Use of Drugs or SURGERY! Learn the secrets in using your own body weight and the law of gravity to INCREASE your muscle mass as you strip away the unwanted fat.

Everyone has a routine; whether it's getting up and going to work, or the way you get ready for bed. A body building routine has to be drafted and thoroughly planned out. Everything from eating habits to how many exercises are performed, and even resting time.

Here are some tips:

You have to make sure you adjust your protein-rich diet as well as your eating habit. Small light meals instead of 3 full-course meals a day would be a normal approach to building your body.

Not only is meal a factor in a body building routine, but the exercise is also a factor. You need strength training excercises that involve both compound and isolated movements.

Nutrition provides a great role in your routine because of the calorie intake. You require more calories than an average person with the same weight due to the protein and energy it takes to excercise.

Your muscle growth occurs only after the exercise, during rest. Without proper rest, your muscles cannot have the opporitunity to heal or increase in size

This is your quick guide to that summer beach body you've always wanted. This manual will cover:

- Body Building Diet Tips
- Body Building Routines
- Body Building Supplements
- Body Building Workouts
- Building Muscle the Natural Way
- Healthy Body Building Nutrition Tips
- How to Build Strength
- Losing Body Fat the Natural Way
- Weight Training Routines
- Weight Training Tips
- And Much Much MORE!!!

Visit the URL above to download this guide and start achieving your weight loss and fitness goals NOW

One Last Thing...

Thank you so much for reading my book. I hope you really liked it. As you probably know, many people look at the reviews on Amazon before they decide to purchase a book. If you liked the book, could you please take a minute to leave a review with your feedback? 60 seconds is all I'm asking for, and it would mean the world to me.

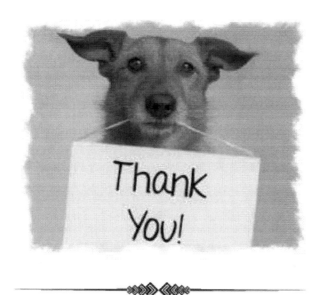

Books by Lars Andersen

The Smoothies for Runners Book

Juices for Runners

Smoothies for Cyclists

Juices for Cyclists

Paleo Diet for Cyclists

Smoothies for Triathletes

Juices for Triathletes

Paleo Diet for Triathletes

Smoothies for Strength

About the Author

Lars Andersen is a sports author, nutritional researcher and fitness enthusiast. In his spare time he participates in competitive running, swimming and cycling events and enjoys hiking with his two border collies.

Lars Andersen

Published by Nordic Standard Publishing

Atlanta, Georgia USA

NORDICSTANDARD
PUBLISHING

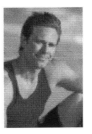

Copyright © 2012 Lars Andersen

Images and Cover by Nordic Standard Publishing

5533894R00041

Printed in Great Britain
by Amazon.co.uk, Ltd.,
Marston Gate.